Dash Diet in a Dash

20 Dash Diet Recipes You Can Make in 15 Minutes or Less

Disclaimer and Terms of Use:

Effort has been made to ensure that the information in this book is accurate and complete, however, the author and the publisher do not warrant the accuracy of the information, text and graphics contained within the book due to the rapidly changing nature of science, research, known and unknown facts and internet. The Author and the publisher do not hold any responsibility for errors, omissions or contrary interpretation of the subject matter herein. This book is presented solely for motivational and informational purposes only.

Table of Contents

Introduction

The DASH (Dietary Approaches to Stop Hypertension) diet was developed as a way to fight or prevent high blood pressure (hypertension) by eating a diet low in sodium and high in potassium, magnesium and calcium. This diet has proven to be as effective as many first-line hypertension drugs, and it also can help prevent other disease such as cancer, heart disease and diabetes.

We all know that it can be difficult to find time to cook healthy meals in the midst of our busy lives. The recipes contained in this book are the quickest, easiest DASH diet recipes around – you can prepare them in 15 minutes or less. There are delicious recipes for breakfast, lunch, dinner and dessert, and they can be easily adapted with other ingredients to create a variety of meals that are good – and good for you.

Breakfast Recipes

It's important to start each day with a healthy breakfast. These recipes are easy to make and delicious.

Apple Cinnamon French Toast

Ingredients:

6 slices whole wheat bread

2 whole eggs or 4 egg whites

½ c. milk

¼ c. unsweetened applesauce

2 Tbsp. white sugar

1 tsp. cinnamon

Cooking spray

Combine the eggs, milk, applesauce, sugar and cinnamon in a large mixing bowl, and whisk until combined. Dip the bread slices into the mixture one at a time, until the bread has absorbed some of the apple cinnamon mixture.

Cook on medium heat on a lightly oiled griddle or skillet until both sides are golden brown. Serve immediately. Makes 6 servings.

Scrambled Eggs with Spinach, Mushrooms and Feta Cheese

Ingredients:

1 whole egg plus 2 egg whites

1 c. chopped fresh spinach

½ c. sliced mushrooms

2 Tbsp. feta cheese

Cooking spray

Pepper to taste

Heat a non-stick pan to medium heat and coat it with cooking spray. Sauté the spinach and mushrooms until the spinach is wilted, about 2-3 minutes.

Whisk the egg, cheese and pepper together, then pour over the vegetables. Cook the eggs, stirring to scramble them, until the eggs are cooked through. Serve hot. Makes 1 serving.

Quick Green Breakfast Smoothie

Ingredients:

1 medium banana (frozen, if preferred)

1 c. spinach leaves, packed

¾ c. frozen mango chunks

½ c. skim milk

¼ c. plain nonfat yogurt

¼ c. whole oats

½ tsp. vanilla extract

Blend milk, oats and yogurt in the blender for about 15 seconds to break up the oats. Add the banana, spinach, mango and vanilla and blend until the mixture is thick and smooth. Serves 1.

Hearty Breakfast Salad

Ingredients:

3 c. water

¾ c. fast-cooking brown rice

¾ c. bulgur wheat

¼ tsp. salt

1 Red Delicious apple

1 Granny Smith apple

1 orange

1 c. raisins

1 c. lowfat vanilla-flavored yogurt

Bring the water and salt to a boil. Add the rice and bulgur wheat, reduce the heat, and cook on low for another 10 minutes. Let the cooked grains sit for another two minutes while you chop the apples and section the orange. Spread the grains out on a cookie sheet to help them cool, then mix the grains, fruits and yogurt together in a large mixing bowl. Makes 6 servings.

(Note: cook and cool the grains the night before for quick prep in the morning.)

No-Bake Granola Bars

Ingredients:

2 ½ c. toasted rice cereal

2 c. old fashioned rolled oats

½ c. brown sugar, packed

½ c. light corn syrup

½ c. peanut butter

½ c. raisins

1 tsp. vanilla extract

Combine the brown sugar and corn syrup in a 1-quart saucepan and bring to a boil. Remove from heat. Stir the peanut butter and vanilla into the sugar mixture and blend until smooth. Put the cereal and raisins into a large mixing bowl and pour the liquid over it, stirring until well mixed.

Put the mixture into a 9 X 13 baking pan and let it cool. Cut into bars. Makes 18 servings.

Banana Split Breakfast

Ingredients:

1 small banana

½ c. granola cereal (substitute oat or corn cereal, if desired)

½ c. low fat yogurt (strawberry or vanilla)

½ c. canned pineapple chunks

2 Tbsp. chopped peanuts

½ tsp. honey

Split the banana lengthwise and put each half in a separate bowl. Split the granola, setting a small amount aside for garnish, and sprinkle over the banana. Spoon the yogurt on top. Add pineapple, peanuts and reserved granola, and drizzle with honey to finish. Serves 2.

Lunch Recipes

Grilled Vegetable Sandwiches

Ingredients:

2 small focaccia rolls, sliced lengthwise

1 c. red bell peppers, sliced

1 small zucchini, sliced

1 small yellow squash, sliced

1 small red onion, sliced

½ c. reduced fat feta cheese

1/8 c. olive oil

3 Tbsp. light mayonnaise

1 Tbsp. lemon juice

3 garlic cloves, minced

Mix the mayonnaise, lemon juice and garlic in a small bowl and refrigerate. Preheat your grill. Brush the sliced vegetables lightly with olive oil and place them on the grill. Cook for 3-4 minutes, then flip and cook them on the other side until cooked through. Set aside on a plate.

Spread the cut sides of the bread with the mayonnaise mixture and sprinkle with the feta cheese. Place them cheese-side up on the grill and cover with lid for about 2-3 minutes, watching to make sure the cheese melts and the bottoms don't burn. Layer the vegetables on top of the cheese. Makes 4 open-face sandwiches.

Tuna Salad with Pasta

Ingredients:

2 c. arugula

1 c. cooked pasta (from 2 oz. dry)

5 oz. can light tuna (packed in water), drained

¼ c. green onion tops, chopped

1 Tbsp. olive oil

1 Tbsp. red wine vinegar

1 Tbsp. parmesan cheese, grated

Pepper to taste

Toss the arugula, pasta, tuna, onions, olive oil and vinegar in a large bowl until mixed. Divide onto two plates and sprinkle with parmesan cheese and pepper. Makes 2 servings.

Curry Tofu Salad

Ingredients:

1 14 oz. package firm, water-packed tofu, drained, patted dry and crumbled

1 c. red grapes, sliced in half

2 celery stalks, diced

½ c. sliced scallions

¼ c. walnuts

3 Tbsp. plain low-fat yogurt

2 Tbsp. light mayonnaise

2 Tbsp. mango chutney

2 tsp. Madras curry powder

¼ tsp. salt

Pepper to taste

Combine the yogurt, mayonnaise, chutney, curry powder, salt and pepper in a large bowl. Make sure the curry powder is completely blended in. Fold in the tofu, grapes, celery, scallions and walnuts. Makes 6 servings.

Pita Pocket Pizzas

Ingredients:

2 pieces whole grain pita bread

½ c. shredded low-salt mozzarella

¼ c. tomato sauce

Assorted vegetables: mushrooms, peppers, onions, zucchini, olives, etc.

Preheat the oven to 350 F (175 C). Split the pita bread halfway around the edge. Spoon in the vegetables, tomato sauce and cheese. Wrap the pitas in aluminum foil and bake until the cheese is melted, about 7-10 minutes. Makes 2 servings.

Egg and Avocado Salad

Ingredients:

4 large hard-boiled eggs, whites and yolks chopped separately

4 hard-boiled egg whites, chopped

1 medium avocado, chopped into ½ inch pieces

1 Tbsp. fat-free plain yogurt

1 Tbsp. light mayonnaise

½ Tbsp. chives, chopped

2 tsp. red wine vinegar

½ tsp. salt

Pepper to taste

6 slices whole wheat bread, toasted

Combine the egg yolks, avocado, yogurt, mayonnaise, chives, vinegar, salt and pepper and mash with a fork until smooth. Add the egg whites and mix until coated. Spoon onto toasted bread and serve as an open-face sandwich. Makes 6 servings.

Dinner

Easy Broccoli Pasta

Ingredients:

12 oz. uncooked pasta

6 ½ c. broccoli florets

¼ c. grated Parmesan or Romano cheese

5 cloves garlic, chopped

2 Tbsp. olive oil, divided

Salt & pepper to taste

Bring a large pot of salted water to a boil. Add the pasta and broccoli and cook until the pasta is al dente. Reserve 1 c. of pasta water and drain the pasta and broccoli.

Return the pot to the stove. Put it on high heat and add 1 Tbsp. of the olive oil. Sauté the garlic until slightly browned. Add the pasta and broccoli, remaining olive oil, cheese, salt and pepper and toss until coated. Add pasta water if necessary to loosen the sauce. Serves 6.

Quick Cranberry Chicken Breasts

Ingredients:

1 lb. boneless skinless chicken breasts

¾ whole cranberry sauce

¼ c. chili sauce

¼ c. apple juice

1 tsp. butter

1 tsp. brown sugar

¼ tsp. black pepper

Pound the chicken to thin it slightly and sprinkle with the black pepper. Melt the butter in a large skillet and brown chicken on both sides. Add the rest of the ingredients and simmer with the lid on for about 15 minutes, or until the chicken is almost cooked through. Remove the lid and let the sauce boil for a little longer until it thickens. Serve with steamed brown rice and vegetables. Serves 4.

Pesto Shrimp Skewers

Ingredients:

1 ½ lbs. jumbo shrimp, peeled and cleaned

Salt & black pepper to taste

7 metal skewers (if you use wood skewers, make sure to soak them first)

For Marinade:

1 c. chopped fresh basil

¼ c. grated Parmesan cheese

3 Tbsp. olive oil

1 clove garlic, peeled

Put the basil, cheese, olive oil, garlic, salt and pepper in a food processor and pulse until smooth. Pour the marinade into a bowl with the raw shrimp and stir to coat. Refrigerate for several hours.

Preheat your grill or grill pan to medium-high heat. Put the shrimp onto the skewers. Spray the grill lightly with cooking spray. Cook the skewers until the shrimp are pink on one side (about 2-3 minutes) then flip them and cook an additional 3-4 minutes until the shrimp are fully cooked. This goes well with salad and brown rice. Serves 7.

Apple Cheddar Quesadillas

Ingredients:

4 medium whole wheat tortillas

1 c. apples, sliced

1 c. grated cheddar cheese

½ c. red pepper, finely chopped

2 Tbsp. minced onion

Lay out two tortillas. Put ¼ of the cheese on each tortilla. Divide the apples, peppers and onion between the two tortillas, the rest of the cheese, and top with the remaining tortillas.

Heat a griddle or skillet to medium heat. Spray lightly with cooking spray and cook the quesadillas until the bottom is golden brown. Flip and continue cooking until the other side is brown and the cheese is melted. Serves 4.

Southwest Sweet Potatoes

Ingredients:

4 medium sweet potatoes

1 1/3 c. reduced-salt black beans, drained

½ c. red pepper, diced

½ c. red onion, diced

½ c. low-fat Mexican cheese blend

½ c. salsa

½ c. fat free Greek yogurt or sour cream.

¼ c. chopped cilantro or scallions

1 tsp. olive oil

1 tsp. low-salt taco seasoning

1 tsp. chili powder

½ tsp. cumin

½ tsp. paprika

Pinch of salt

Poke holes in the sweet potatoes with a fork and cook them in your microwave for 8-10 minutes on high, until they are cooked through. Blend the yogurt and taco seasoning and set aside. While the potatoes are cooking, heat the olive oil in a skillet and cook the onions, peppers, chili powder, cumin and salt until the vegetables are soft and slightly caramelized. Add the black beans and heat through.

Slice the sweet potatoes lengthwise and divide the cheese, black bean mixture, yogurt mixture and salsa between them. Serves 4.

Desserts

Easy Apple Cinnamon Shake

Ingredients:

2 c. low-fat vanilla ice cream

1 c. unsweetened applesauce

1 c. skim milk

¼ tsp. cinnamon

Put the ice cream, applesauce and cinnamon in a blender and combine. Add the skim milk and continue to blend until smooth. Makes 4 servings.

Trifle with Strawberries and Pears

Ingredients:

2 c. strawberries, hulled and sliced

2 pears, peeled, cored and thinly sliced

½ 9" angel food cake, cubed

3 c. vanilla or lemon flavored low-fat yogurt

2 Tbsp. lemon juice

2 Tbsp. orange juice

2 Tbsp. honey

½ tsp. almond extract, optional

Toss the pears with the lemon juice and the strawberries with the almond extract. Combine the orange juice and honey.

In a large (2 – 2 ½ qt. bowl) layer as follows:

- One third of cake
- Sprinkle with 1 Tbsp. of orange juice and honey mixture
- 1 c. yogurt
- 1 c. strawberry slices
- 1 c. pear slices

Repeat the layers, then top with the remaining cake sprinkled with orange juice and the final cup of yogurt. This can be made in advance and refrigerated for 1-4 hours. Top with pear slices and mint. Serves 10.

Speedy Chocolate Pudding

2 c. skim milk

1/3 c. chocolate chips

3 Tbsp. cornstarch

2 Tbsp. cocoa powder

2 Tbsp. sugar

½ tsp. vanilla extract

Pinch of salt

Mix the cornstarch, cocoa powder, sugar and salt in a saucepan until combined. Whisk in the milk. Heat the mixture on medium until it thickens and is just starting to bubble. Remove from the heat and stir in the chocolate chips and vanilla until the chips melt. Spoon the mixture into 4 individual serving dishes and cover with plastic wrap (make sure the wrap touches the pudding to prevent a skin from forming) and refrigerate until set. Serves 4.

Baked Apples with Coconut and Apricots

Ingredients:

4 Golden Delicious apples

½ c. orange juice

¼ c. flaked coconut

¼ c. dried apricots, chopped

2 Tbsp. brown sugar

2 tsp. grated orange zest

Peel the top third of the apples, core them and place them in a microwave-safe dish. Combine the flaked coconut, apricots and orange zest and spoon the mixture into the center of the apples. Combine the brown sugar and orange juice and pour it over the top. Cover with (vented) plastic wrap and microwave on high for 7-8 minutes or until the apples are soft.